Fibromyalgia Journey:

A Guide To Building Resilience

Dr. Martin Harper

1

This Book Is Dedicated To My lovely wife Sandra and my son Jacob. You have both been very instrumental to my journey in this medical field.

TABLE OF CONTENTS

CHAPTER ONE: UNDERSTANDING FIBROMYALGIA

Introduction to Fibromyalgia: definition, prevalence, and historical context.

Fibromyalgia is a complex and often misunderstood chronic condition that profoundly affects the lives of those who experience it. At its core, fibromyalgia is characterized by widespread musculoskeletal pain, accompanied by fatigue, sleep disturbances, and cognitive challenges. While the exact cause remains elusive, the condition is thought to involve a heightened response to pain signals in the brain and changes in neurotransmitter levels.

The prevalence of fibromyalgia is significant, with estimates suggesting millions of individuals worldwide are affected. However, pinning down an accurate number is challenging, as many cases go undiagnosed or are misdiagnosed due to the varied and sometimes elusive nature of its symptoms. Fibromyalgia can impact anyone, regardless of age or gender, but it is most commonly diagnosed in middle-aged individuals, particularly women.

To understand the impact of fibromyalgia, it's crucial to delve into its historical context. While the term "fibromyalgia" was coined relatively recently in the late 20th century, the condition's history can be traced back centuries. In the 19th century, physicians described a cluster of symptoms resembling fibromyalgia under different names, such as muscular rheumatism. However, it wasn't until the late 20th century that medical professionals recognized fibromyalgia as a distinct clinical entity.

Historically, fibromyalgia patients often faced skepticism within the medical community due to the absence of visible signs of illness and the subjective nature of pain. This lack of understanding contributed to a delayed recognition of fibromyalgia as a legitimate health concern. Over the years, advancements in medical research and a growing body of scientific evidence have validated the experiences of individuals with fibromyalgia, leading to increased awareness and improved diagnostic criteria.

The diagnostic journey for fibromyalgia is often protracted and challenging. It involves a thorough examination of symptoms, often ruling out other conditions with similar presentations. The American College of Rheumatology criteria, established in 1990 and updated in 2010, play a pivotal role in diagnosing fibromyalgia by assessing the extent of pain and tenderness in specific body regions.

Despite the progress in understanding and diagnosing fibromyalgia, misconceptions persist. Some may perceive it as merely a manifestation of psychological distress or dismiss it as "just aches and pains." However, the reality is far more complex. Fibromyalgia not only affects physical well-being but also has a profound impact on mental health and overall quality of life.

Overview of symptoms and how they impact daily life.

Fibromyalgia is a multifaceted condition that manifests through a diverse array of symptoms, creating a profound impact on the daily lives of those affected. Understanding these symptoms is crucial for individuals, caregivers, and healthcare professionals alike to navigate the challenges associated with fibromyalgia.

The hallmark symptom of fibromyalgia is widespread musculoskeletal pain, often described as a deep, persistent ache. This pain is not limited to a specific area but is rather dispersed throughout the body, affecting muscles, tendons, and ligaments. It tends to be accompanied by heightened sensitivity to pressure, with even mild touch causing discomfort—a phenomenon known as allodynia.

Fatigue is another prevalent symptom, extending beyond ordinary tiredness. Individuals with fibromyalgia often experience a persistent, overwhelming sense of exhaustion, even after a full night's sleep. This fatigue can significantly impact daily activities, making routine tasks challenging and contributing to a sense of overall malaise.

Sleep disturbances are common among those with fibromyalgia, further exacerbating the fatigue they experience. Despite spending adequate time in bed, individuals may struggle with achieving restorative sleep due to disruptions in sleep patterns, such as frequent awakenings or difficulty reaching deep sleep stages. The interplay between pain and sleep disturbances creates a vicious cycle, with each exacerbating the other.

Cognitive difficulties, often referred to as "fibro fog," present another layer of challenges. Individuals may experience issues with concentration, memory, and mental clarity. This cognitive dysfunction can impact work performance, daily decision-making, and overall quality of life.

Beyond these primary symptoms, fibromyalgia often coexists with a range of secondary symptoms that vary from person to person. These may include headaches, irritable bowel syndrome (IBS), temporomandibular joint (TMJ) disorders, and heightened sensitivity to stimuli such as light, noise, and temperature. The combination of these symptoms creates a complex and individualized experience of fibromyalgia for each affected person.

The impact of fibromyalgia on daily life is profound, affecting various aspects of an individual's well-being. Employment may become challenging due to fatigue, cognitive difficulties, and the unpredictability of symptom flare-ups. Maintaining relationships can be strained as individuals navigate the emotional toll of living with chronic pain and fatigue. Additionally, participating in social activities or hobbies may be limited, further impacting one's sense of fulfillment and connection.

The unpredictable nature of fibromyalgia symptoms adds an additional layer of complexity to daily life. Individuals may face the uncertainty of not knowing when a flare-up will occur or how severe it will be. This uncertainty can contribute to anxiety and stress, further exacerbating the symptoms and creating a cyclical pattern of physical and emotional challenges.

In the upcoming chapters, we'll delve into the intricacies of fibromyalgia, exploring potential causes, the diagnostic process, available treatments, and daily strategies for managing this challenging condition. By gaining a comprehensive understanding, we aim to support those living with fibromyalgia, dispel misconceptions, and explore a range of strategies, from medical interventions to lifestyle adjustments, to improve overall quality of life for individuals facing this complex condition.

CHAPTER TWO: UNRAVELING THE CAUSES

Exploration of potential causes and triggers of fibromyalgia

The etiology of fibromyalgia remains a subject of ongoing research and debate within the medical community. While a definitive cause has yet to be identified, several factors and potential triggers have been explored to better understand the complex nature of this chronic condition.

Genetic predisposition is one avenue of investigation into the origins of fibromyalgia. Studies have suggested a familial clustering of fibromyalgia cases, indicating a potential genetic component. Research is ongoing to identify specific genes associated with an increased susceptibility to fibromyalgia, but the interplay between genetics and environmental factors remains intricate.

Environmental factors, including physical and emotional stressors, are considered potential triggers for fibromyalgia onset or exacerbation. Traumatic events, such as accidents, surgeries, or emotional distress, have been linked to the development of fibromyalgia symptoms in some individuals. The stress response may play a role in triggering physiological changes that contribute to the amplification of pain signals in the central nervous system.

Infections and illnesses are also being explored as potential triggers for fibromyalgia. Some individuals report the onset of fibromyalgia symptoms following infections, leading researchers to investigate the connection between immune system dysfunction and the development of the condition. Chronic infections, such as viral or bacterial infections, may contribute to the dysregulation of the immune response, impacting the nervous system and potentially triggering fibromyalgia symptoms.

Neurotransmitter imbalances, particularly involving serotonin and norepinephrine, have been implicated in fibromyalgia. These chemical messengers play a crucial role in pain modulation, mood regulation, and sleep patterns. Research suggests that an imbalance in these neurotransmitters may contribute to the heightened pain sensitivity, sleep disturbances, and mood disorders often observed in individuals with fibromyalgia.

Central sensitization, a process wherein the central nervous system becomes hypersensitive to pain signals, is a key aspect of fibromyalgia pathology. It is believed that repeated nerve stimulation, whether from injuries, infections, or other factors, can lead to changes in the brain and spinal cord, amplifying pain signals. This central sensitization may contribute to the widespread and persistent pain experienced by individuals with fibromyalgia.

Hormonal factors, particularly disturbances in the hypothalamic-pituitary-adrenal (HPA) axis, are also under scrutiny. The HPA axis plays a crucial role in the body's stress response and hormone regulation. Dysregulation of this axis has been observed in some individuals with fibromyalgia and may contribute to the symptoms associated with the condition.

It's important to note that fibromyalgia is a heterogeneous condition, and the interplay of these potential causes may vary from person to person. Furthermore, these factors are not necessarily mutually exclusive, and it is likely that a combination of genetic, environmental, and physiological elements contributes to the development and persistence of fibromyalgia symptoms.

Discussion on genetic factors, environmental influences, and the role of stress.

Understanding the origins of fibromyalgia requires a comprehensive examination of genetic factors, environmental influences, and the role of stress. These interconnected elements contribute to the complex tapestry of fibromyalgia, shaping its onset, progression, and symptomatology. Delving into each of these components provides insight into the intricate mechanisms underlying this chronic condition.

Genetic Factors:
The exploration of genetic factors in fibromyalgia is a multifaceted endeavor. While no single gene has been identified as the sole culprit, familial aggregation studies suggest a genetic predisposition. Research indicates that individuals with a family history of fibromyalgia are more likely to develop the condition themselves, hinting at a hereditary component.

Twin studies have also played a role in unraveling the genetic underpinnings of fibromyalgia. Identical twins, who share nearly identical genetic makeup, are more likely to both have fibromyalgia compared to non-identical twins. This supports the notion that genetics contribute to susceptibility.

However, the genetic landscape of fibromyalgia is far from straightforward. It involves an intricate interplay of multiple genes, each potentially contributing a small effect. The search for specific genetic markers associated with fibromyalgia susceptibility is ongoing, with researchers exploring various candidate genes linked to pain perception, neurotransmitter regulation, and immune system function.

Moreover, genetic factors alone do not determine fibromyalgia development. Environmental influences and lifestyle factors play a crucial role in whether genetic predispositions manifest into clinical symptoms. Understanding these genetic factors is a critical step, but it is equally important to explore how they interact with the environment.

Environmental Influences:
Environmental factors encompass a broad range of external elements that can influence the development and exacerbation of fibromyalgia. These include physical, psychological, and social aspects of an individual's surroundings.

Traumatic events, both physical and emotional, have been identified as potential triggers for fibromyalgia. Injuries from accidents or surgeries may serve as catalysts for the onset of symptoms. Similarly, emotional stressors, such as the loss of a loved one or chronic psychological stress, have been linked to the development and exacerbation of fibromyalgia symptoms. The intricate connection between the mind and body underscores the importance of considering psychological well-being in the context of fibromyalgia.

Chronic infections have also been implicated as environmental triggers. Some individuals report the onset of fibromyalgia symptoms following infections, suggesting a potential link between immune system dysfunction and fibromyalgia. The body's response to infections, particularly viral or bacterial, may contribute to the dysregulation of the immune response, further impacting the nervous system and potentially triggering fibromyalgia symptoms.

Furthermore, lifestyle factors such as diet, physical activity, and sleep patterns can influence fibromyalgia. Poor sleep quality, in particular, is both a symptom and a potential exacerbating factor, creating a challenging cycle where disturbed sleep contributes to symptoms and vice versa.

The Role of Stress:
Stress, whether physical or psychological, is a pervasive factor in the landscape of fibromyalgia. The intricate relationship between stress and fibromyalgia symptoms is bidirectional, with stress both triggering and being exacerbated by the condition.

The body's stress response involves the activation of the hypothalamic-pituitary-adrenal (HPA) axis, which releases stress hormones like cortisol. Dysregulation of the HPA axis has been observed in fibromyalgia patients, suggesting a connection between abnormal stress responses and the condition.

Chronic stress, whether due to ongoing life challenges or a traumatic event, can contribute to the onset of fibromyalgia symptoms. The physiological changes induced by stress, including heightened sensitivity to pain signals and immune system dysregulation, may play a role in the amplification of fibromyalgia symptoms.

Conversely, the symptoms of fibromyalgia themselves, particularly chronic pain and fatigue, create a persistent state of stress for affected individuals. The daily challenges of managing pain, coping with fatigue, and navigating the unpredictability of symptoms contribute to an ongoing stress burden.

The relationship between stress and fibromyalgia is further complicated by the individual variability in stress responses. What may be a significant stressor for one person may not have the same impact on another. Additionally, the coping mechanisms individuals employ to manage stress can influence the course of fibromyalgia.

Interconnected Dynamics:
It's crucial to recognize the interconnected dynamics of genetic factors, environmental influences, and stress in the context of fibromyalgia. These elements do not operate in isolation but rather influence each other in intricate ways.

Genetic predispositions may create vulnerability to environmental triggers, and the body's stress response can modulate how these genetic factors manifest. For example, a person with a genetic predisposition to fibromyalgia may not develop symptoms unless exposed to certain environmental stressors.

Moreover, the impact of stress is not uniform across all individuals with fibromyalgia. Some may find that stress exacerbates their symptoms significantly, while others may not perceive a direct correlation. The variability in individual experiences underscores the complexity of fibromyalgia as a condition shaped by both intrinsic and extrinsic factors.

Understanding the interconnected dynamics involves recognizing that fibromyalgia is a heterogeneous condition with diverse manifestations. The intricate interplay of genetic, environmental, and stress-related factors contributes to the variability in symptomatology and the individualized nature of the fibromyalgia experience.

Chapter 3: DIAGNOSING FIBROMYALGIA

Explanation of the diagnostic process, highlighting the challenges and common misconceptions.

The diagnostic process for fibromyalgia is a complex journey that involves a careful evaluation of symptoms, ruling out other potential causes, and considering established criteria. Despite advancements in understanding the condition, challenges and misconceptions persist, contributing to delays in diagnosis and sometimes, misinterpretations of the patient's experience.

Clinical Criteria and Challenges:

The diagnostic criteria for fibromyalgia have evolved over time. The American College of Rheumatology (ACR) introduced criteria in 1990 that focused on tender points—specific areas on the body that are sensitive to pressure. However, recognizing the limitations of this approach, the ACR updated the criteria in 2010 to shift the emphasis from tender points to a more comprehensive evaluation of symptoms.

The 2010 criteria include widespread pain index (WPI) and symptom severity (SS) scales. WPI assesses pain across 19 different body areas, while SS evaluates the severity of other symptoms such as fatigue, cognitive difficulties, and sleep disturbances. To meet the criteria, a patient should have widespread pain for at least three months and a certain score on the WPI and SS scales.

Despite these criteria, challenges persist. Some healthcare providers may not be familiar with the updated guidelines, leading to the continued use of older, more restrictive criteria. This can result in

27

misdiagnosis or delayed diagnosis for individuals who meet the newer, more inclusive standards.

Additionally, the subjective nature of pain poses challenges. Pain is a deeply personal experience, and patients may struggle to convey the extent and impact of their symptoms accurately. This subjectivity can contribute to skepticism from healthcare professionals who may rely on more tangible, objective evidence for diagnosis.

The Complexity of Symptomatology: Fibromyalgia is characterized by a diverse array of symptoms beyond pain, including fatigue, sleep disturbances, cognitive difficulties, and mood disorders. The challenge lies in the variability and overlap of these symptoms with other conditions, making diagnosis more intricate.

Common misconceptions about fibromyalgia may arise due to the diversity of symptoms. Some healthcare providers may attribute the symptoms to other conditions or dismiss them as psychosomatic. The complex interplay of physical and psychological aspects in fibromyalgia can contribute to misunderstandings, leading to delayed or inaccurate diagnoses.

Moreover, the fluctuating nature of fibromyalgia symptoms adds another layer of complexity. Symptoms may wax and wane, making it challenging for healthcare providers to capture the full extent of the patient's experience during a single appointment. This variability can contribute to the misconception that symptoms are not consistent or severe enough to warrant a fibromyalgia diagnosis.

Overcoming Misconceptions:
Addressing misconceptions requires an integrated and multidisciplinary approach. Healthcare providers need to be educated on the evolving diagnostic criteria and the diverse symptomatology of fibromyalgia. Increased awareness and training can lead to more accurate and timely diagnoses, minimizing the risk of misinterpretation.

Patients, too, play a crucial role in the diagnostic process. Open communication about symptoms, their impact on daily life, and a willingness to advocate for themselves can help bridge the gap between subjective experiences and clinical assessments. Keeping a detailed symptom journal can provide healthcare providers with valuable insights into the patterns and severity of symptoms over time.

Moreover, fostering a collaborative relationship between patients and healthcare providers is essential. A holistic approach that considers both physical and psychological aspects of fibromyalgia can contribute to a more accurate diagnosis and tailored treatment plan.

The diagnostic process for fibromyalgia is intricate, involving a nuanced evaluation of symptoms and an understanding of evolving criteria. Challenges and misconceptions persist, but with increased awareness, education, and a collaborative approach between patients and healthcare providers, the path to an accurate diagnosis can be navigated more effectively. Recognizing fibromyalgia as a complex condition with diverse manifestations is crucial for providing individuals with the support and understanding they need on their healthcare journey.

Insights into the importance of a multidisciplinary approach in diagnosis.

The importance of a multidisciplinary approach in the diagnosis of fibromyalgia cannot be overstated. Given the complex nature of the condition, which encompasses a spectrum of symptoms affecting various aspects of an individual's health, a collaborative effort among healthcare professionals from different specialties is essential for accurate diagnosis and effective management.

Comprehensive Symptom Evaluation: Fibromyalgia extends beyond the traditional boundaries of a single medical specialty.

31

While rheumatologists often play a key role in diagnosing fibromyalgia, the condition's diverse symptomatology requires insights from various disciplines. A multidisciplinary team may include rheumatologists, neurologists, sleep specialists, psychologists, and pain management experts. Each specialist brings a unique perspective, contributing to a more comprehensive evaluation of the patient's symptoms.

Addressing Physical and Psychological Components:
Fibromyalgia is characterized by the interplay between physical and psychological aspects. Pain, fatigue, and sleep disturbances are intertwined with emotional well-being and cognitive functioning. A multidisciplinary approach recognizes the interconnected nature of these components, ensuring that both physical and psychological aspects are thoroughly assessed.

Psychologists or mental health professionals are integral members of the multidisciplinary team, as they can evaluate the impact of fibromyalgia on a patient's mental health, assess coping mechanisms, and provide strategies for managing stress. This holistic approach acknowledges that addressing the psychological aspects of fibromyalgia is crucial for comprehensive care.

Improving Accuracy in Diagnosis:
The collaboration of specialists in a multidisciplinary team enhances the accuracy of the diagnostic process. Different perspectives and expertise contribute to a more thorough evaluation of symptoms, reducing the risk of misdiagnosis or overlooking crucial aspects of the condition. A multidisciplinary team is better equipped to navigate the complexity of fibromyalgia, considering its diverse manifestations and ensuring that all relevant factors are taken into account.

Tailoring Treatment Plans:
Once a fibromyalgia diagnosis is established, a multidisciplinary approach becomes equally essential in crafting personalized treatment plans. Different

specialists can contribute to the development of strategies that address specific aspects of the condition. For instance, a rheumatologist may focus on pain management, a sleep specialist on improving sleep quality, and a psychologist on addressing emotional well-being. This tailored approach recognizes that fibromyalgia is not a one-size-fits-all condition, and treatment plans should be as diverse as the symptoms themselves.

Enhancing Patient Support and Education: A multidisciplinary team not only contributes to accurate diagnosis and effective treatment but also plays a pivotal role in supporting and educating patients. Comprehensive patient education, provided by healthcare professionals from various disciplines, can empower individuals with fibromyalgia to better understand and manage their condition. Furthermore, the collaborative support of a multidisciplinary team can help patients navigate the challenges of living with fibromyalgia and provide a sense of validation for their experiences.

Building a Collaborative Network: Establishing a collaborative network of healthcare professionals fosters ongoing communication and coordination of care. Regular information exchange between specialists ensures that any changes in the patient's condition are promptly addressed, leading to a more proactive and responsive approach to managing fibromyalgia.

A multidisciplinary approach is indispensable in the diagnosis and management of fibromyalgia. This collaborative model acknowledges the complexity of the condition, addresses both physical and psychological components, enhances diagnostic accuracy, tailors treatment plans, and provides comprehensive support for individuals living with fibromyalgia. By embracing a multidisciplinary perspective, healthcare providers can offer more effective and holistic care, ultimately improving the quality of life for those affected by this challenging condition.

Chapter 4: Navigating the Medical Landscape

Comprehensive overview of available treatments, from medications to alternative therapies.

The treatment landscape for fibromyalgia is multifaceted, involving a combination of medications, lifestyle modifications, and alternative therapies. Given the diverse and individualized nature of fibromyalgia symptoms, a comprehensive approach that addresses various aspects of the condition is often necessary to improve overall well-being.

Medications:
1. Pain Relievers: Over-the-counter pain relievers like acetaminophen or nonsteroidal

anti-inflammatory drugs (NSAIDs) may be recommended for managing pain. However, their efficacy for fibromyalgia is limited, and prescription medications are often considered for more significant relief.

2. Antidepressants: Certain antidepressants, such as amitriptyline, duloxetine, and milnacipran, have been found to be effective in managing fibromyalgia symptoms. They can help alleviate pain, improve sleep, and address mood disturbances.

3. Anticonvulsants: Medications like pregabalin and gabapentin, originally developed to treat seizures, have shown efficacy in reducing fibromyalgia-related pain.

Lifestyle Modifications:

1. Regular Exercise: Physical activity is a cornerstone of fibromyalgia management. Low-impact exercises such as walking, swimming, or gentle yoga can help improve flexibility, reduce pain, and enhance overall well-being.

2. Sleep Hygiene: Establishing good sleep habits is crucial for managing fibromyalgia symptoms. Maintaining a consistent sleep

schedule, creating a comfortable sleep environment, and practicing relaxation techniques can contribute to better sleep quality.

3. Stress Management: Stress can exacerbate fibromyalgia symptoms, so stress-reduction techniques like mindfulness, meditation, and deep breathing exercises can be beneficial.

Physical Therapy:
Physical therapy is often recommended to help manage pain and improve function. Therapists may use techniques such as massage, stretching, and strengthening exercises tailored to the individual's needs. Hydrotherapy or aquatic exercise can also be particularly beneficial.

Cognitive-Behavioral Therapy (CBT):
CBT is a psychological therapy that focuses on changing negative thought patterns and behaviors. It has been shown to be effective in managing fibromyalgia by addressing the psychological aspects of the condition, such as coping with pain and improving overall mental well-being.

Acupuncture:
Acupuncture involves the insertion of thin needles into specific points on the body. Some individuals with fibromyalgia report relief from pain and improved sleep after acupuncture sessions. While research on acupuncture for fibromyalgia is mixed, some find it to be a complementary therapy that provides relief.

Chiropractic Care:
Chiropractic treatment involves spinal adjustments and manipulations to alleviate pain and improve joint function. Some individuals with fibromyalgia find relief from chiropractic care, although its effectiveness can vary.

Mind-Body Practices:
Mind-body practices, such as tai chi and qigong, combine physical movements with mindfulness and deep breathing. These practices can enhance flexibility, reduce stress, and improve overall well-being for individuals with fibromyalgia.

Dietary Interventions:

While no specific diet has been proven to cure fibromyalgia, some individuals report symptom improvement with dietary changes. Adopting an anti-inflammatory diet, which includes whole foods, fruits, vegetables, and omega-3 fatty acids, may help reduce symptoms for some individuals.

Medication Management:
In addition to medications targeting pain and other symptoms, individuals with fibromyalgia may benefit from a comprehensive approach to medication management. This includes coordinating medications to address different aspects of the condition, managing side effects, and regularly reassessing the treatment plan based on the individual's response.

Patient Education and Support:
Educating individuals about fibromyalgia, its management strategies, and providing ongoing support are crucial components of treatment. Support groups, both online and in-person, can offer a sense of community and understanding for individuals navigating the challenges of fibromyalgia.

The treatment of fibromyalgia requires a multifaceted approach that addresses physical, psychological, and lifestyle aspects. Medications, alternative therapies, and lifestyle modifications can be combined based on the individual's needs, preferences, and response to treatment. A collaborative and patient-centered approach involving healthcare providers, physical therapists, mental health professionals, and individuals with fibromyalgia is essential for optimizing treatment outcomes and improving overall quality of life.

Examination of the latest medical research and emerging treatments.

Below is a general overview of some trends and areas of interest in the latest medical research and emerging treatments for fibromyalgia. However, it's crucial to note that the field of medical research is continually evolving, and new developments may have occurred since then.

1. Neurotransmitter Modulators:
Research continues to explore medications that target neurotransmitter imbalances associated with fibromyalgia. Drugs affecting glutamate, serotonin, and norepinephrine receptors are under investigation. For example, novel formulations of existing drugs or new medications that modulate these neurotransmitters are being explored for their potential efficacy in managing fibromyalgia symptoms.

2. Immune System Modulation:
Some studies are investigating the role of the immune system in fibromyalgia. Immunomodulatory therapies, including medications traditionally used for autoimmune conditions, are being explored to understand their potential impact on fibromyalgia symptoms. This reflects a growing recognition of the immune system's involvement in the development and persistence of fibromyalgia.

3. Gut Microbiome and Diet:

Research has shown a potential link between the gut microbiome and fibromyalgia symptoms. Emerging studies explore the impact of diet, probiotics, and interventions targeting the gut microbiota in managing fibromyalgia. Understanding the gut-brain connection and its influence on symptomatology may pave the way for personalized dietary interventions.

4. Non-Pharmacological Approaches:
Advancements in non-pharmacological interventions are gaining attention. High-frequency transcranial magnetic stimulation (TMS) is one such technique being explored for its potential in alleviating pain and improving overall function in individuals with fibromyalgia. Cognitive training and virtual reality-based therapies are also emerging as novel approaches in managing fibromyalgia-related cognitive dysfunction.

5. Targeted Pain Therapies:
Research is investigating targeted pain therapies that focus on specific pain pathways. This includes medications that modulate ion channels involved in pain

signaling. Drugs targeting specific receptors or neural pathways associated with pain perception are being studied to develop more precise and effective pain management strategies.

6. Precision Medicine:
Advancements in understanding the genetic and molecular underpinnings of fibromyalgia are paving the way for precision medicine approaches. Tailoring treatments based on an individual's genetic makeup, biomarkers, and specific symptomatology is an area of active exploration. This personalized approach aims to optimize treatment outcomes and reduce the trial-and-error nature of fibromyalgia management.

7. Digital Health Interventions:
The integration of digital health technologies is becoming more prominent. Mobile applications, wearables, and telehealth platforms are being utilized to monitor symptoms, deliver targeted interventions, and enhance patient-provider communication. These technologies aim to

empower individuals with fibromyalgia to actively participate in their care and provide healthcare professionals with real-time data for more informed decision-making.

It's important to note that while these areas show promise, not all emerging treatments may progress to widespread clinical use. Clinical trials are ongoing, and rigorous research is necessary to validate the safety and efficacy of these potential interventions.

If interested in the latest developments in fibromyalgia research, you should attend scientific conferences, and stay informed through reliable healthcare sources for the most up-to-date information.

Chapter 5: Living with Fibromyalgia: Daily Strategies

Practical advice for managing symptoms in daily life.

Managing fibromyalgia symptoms in daily life involves a combination of lifestyle adjustments, self-care practices, and a proactive approach to overall well-being. Here is practical advice to help navigate the challenges associated with fibromyalgia:

1. Establish a Consistent Sleep Routine: Prioritize good sleep hygiene by maintaining a regular sleep schedule. Create a calming bedtime routine, ensure a comfortable sleep environment, and avoid stimulants like caffeine or electronic devices close to bedtime. Quality sleep is crucial for

managing fatigue and overall symptom relief.

2. Engage in Gentle Exercise:
Incorporate low-impact exercises into your routine, such as walking, swimming, or gentle yoga. Regular physical activity can help improve flexibility, reduce pain, and enhance overall well-being. Start with short sessions and gradually increase the duration as tolerated.

3. Pace Yourself:
Practice pacing to manage energy levels. Break tasks into smaller, manageable segments, and take breaks between activities. Avoid overexertion and listen to your body's signals to prevent symptom flare-ups.

4. Manage Stress:
Develop stress management techniques, such as deep breathing exercises, meditation, or mindfulness. Stress can exacerbate fibromyalgia symptoms, so finding effective coping mechanisms is

essential. Consider activities that promote relaxation and emotional well-being.

5. Maintain a Balanced Diet:
Adopt a healthy, well-balanced diet rich in whole foods, fruits, vegetables, and lean proteins. Stay hydrated and be mindful of how certain foods may impact your symptoms. Some individuals find relief by reducing their intake of processed foods, caffeine, and artificial additives.

6. Prioritize Mental Health:
Addressing the psychological aspects of fibromyalgia is crucial. Consider counseling or therapy, such as cognitive-behavioral therapy (CBT), to develop coping strategies, manage stress, and improve overall mental well-being. Connect with support groups to share experiences and gain insights from others facing similar challenges.

7. Create an Ergonomic Environment:
Optimize your living and working spaces to reduce physical strain. Use ergonomic furniture, arrange workstations to support good posture, and make adjustments to

minimize discomfort. Pay attention to ergonomics in daily activities to prevent unnecessary stress on your body.

8. Temperature Regulation:
Be mindful of temperature extremes, as both heat and cold can impact fibromyalgia symptoms. Dress in layers to manage temperature changes, use heating pads or cold packs as needed, and consider the climate when planning activities.

9. Stay Hydrated:
Proper hydration is essential for overall health. Drink an adequate amount of water throughout the day to support bodily functions. Dehydration can contribute to fatigue and muscle stiffness, so be mindful of your fluid intake.

10. Communicate with Healthcare Providers:
Maintain open communication with your healthcare team. Discuss changes in symptoms, treatment effectiveness, and any concerns you may have. Collaborate with your healthcare providers to adjust your

treatment plan as needed and explore new interventions or therapies.

11. Plan for Flare-Ups:
Acknowledge that flare-ups may occur, and have a plan in place for managing them. Consider strategies such as rest, gentle stretching, and pain management techniques. Having a proactive approach to flare-ups can help minimize their impact on your daily life.

12. Keep a Symptom Journal:
Track your symptoms, activities, and any potential triggers in a journal. This can provide valuable insights for both you and your healthcare team. Identifying patterns may help in making informed decisions about lifestyle adjustments and treatment strategies.

Remember that managing fibromyalgia is an ongoing process, and individual responses to strategies may vary. It's essential to tailor these practical tips to your specific needs and consult with your healthcare providers for personalized advice and guidance.

Tips for maintaining a healthy lifestyle, including sleep hygiene, nutrition, and exercise.

Maintaining a healthy lifestyle is crucial for individuals with fibromyalgia, as it can positively impact overall well-being and help manage symptoms effectively. Here's a more detailed exploration of tips for maintaining a healthy lifestyle, focusing on sleep hygiene, nutrition, and exercise:

1. Sleep Hygiene:

 Consistent Sleep Schedule: Establish a regular sleep-wake schedule by going to bed and waking up at the same time every day, even on weekends. Consistency helps regulate your body's internal clock.

 Create a Relaxing Bedtime Routine: Develop a calming pre-sleep routine to signal to your body that it's time to wind down. This could include activities like reading a book, taking a warm bath, or practicing relaxation exercises.

Optimize Sleep Environment: Ensure your sleep environment is conducive to rest. Keep the bedroom dark, quiet, and cool. Invest in a comfortable mattress and pillows to support quality sleep.

Limit Stimulants: Avoid stimulants such as caffeine and nicotine close to bedtime, as they can interfere with sleep. Consider establishing a cutoff time for consuming these substances in the afternoon.

Manage Screen Time: Limit exposure to screens, including smartphones, tablets, and computers, before bedtime. The blue light emitted from screens can disrupt the production of the sleep hormone melatonin.

Address Sleep Disorders: If you experience sleep disorders like insomnia or sleep apnea, consult with your healthcare provider for appropriate interventions. Treating underlying sleep issues is crucial for managing fibromyalgia symptoms.

2. Nutrition:

Balanced Diet: Emphasize a balanced diet rich in fruits, vegetables, whole grains, lean proteins, and healthy fats. These nutrient-dense foods provide essential vitamins and minerals that support overall health.

Hydration: Stay well-hydrated by drinking an adequate amount of water throughout the day. Dehydration can contribute to fatigue and muscle stiffness, common symptoms of fibromyalgia.

Meal Timing: Aim for regular and balanced meals. Eating smaller, frequent meals throughout the day may help stabilize energy levels and prevent fluctuations in blood sugar.

Omega-3 Fatty Acids: Include sources of omega-3 fatty acids, such as fatty fish (salmon, mackerel), flaxseeds, and walnuts. Omega-3s have anti-inflammatory properties that may benefit individuals with fibromyalgia.

Limit Processed Foods: Minimize the intake of processed foods, refined sugars, and artificial additives. These can contribute to inflammation and may negatively impact symptoms.

Individualized Approach: Consider working with a registered dietitian to develop an individualized nutrition plan. Some individuals may find relief by identifying and avoiding specific trigger foods.

3. Exercise:

Low-Impact Activities: Engage in low-impact exercises that are gentle on the joints and muscles. Swimming, walking, biking, and tai chi are examples of activities that can be well-tolerated by individuals with fibromyalgia.

Gradual Progression: Start with short durations of exercise and gradually increase intensity and duration as tolerated. Overexertion can lead to symptom flare-ups, so it's important to pace yourself.

Strength Training: Include strength training exercises to improve muscle strength and support joint function. Begin with light weights and focus on proper form to prevent injury.

Flexibility Exercises: Incorporate stretching and flexibility exercises to enhance range of motion and reduce muscle stiffness. Yoga or gentle stretching routines can be beneficial.

Aerobic Exercise: Include aerobic exercises to improve cardiovascular health. Even short sessions of brisk walking can contribute to overall fitness.

Listen to Your Body: Pay attention to your body's signals and adjust your exercise routine accordingly. If you experience increased pain or fatigue, consider modifying activities or incorporating more rest days.

Additional Tips for a Healthy Lifestyle:

Stress Management: Practice stress management techniques such as deep breathing, meditation, or mindfulness. Chronic stress can exacerbate fibromyalgia symptoms, so finding effective coping strategies is crucial.

Social Connection: Maintain social connections and seek support from friends, family, or support groups. Social engagement can positively impact mental well-being and provide a sense of community.

Mind-Body Practices: Explore mind-body practices like meditation, biofeedback, or guided imagery. These techniques can help manage pain, reduce stress, and improve overall quality of life.

Consult with Healthcare Providers: Regularly communicate with your healthcare team about your symptoms, lifestyle changes, and treatment plan. Collaborate on adjustments to optimize your overall care.

Remember that adopting a healthy lifestyle is a gradual process, and individual responses may vary. It's essential to tailor these tips to your unique needs and consult with healthcare providers for personalized guidance. Regularly reassessing and adjusting your approach based on your experiences can contribute to ongoing improvements in your overall health and well-being.

Chapter 6: Emotional Well-being

Exploration of the emotional impact of fibromyalgia.

The emotional impact of fibromyalgia is significant and multifaceted, affecting various aspects of an individual's mental well-being. Living with a chronic condition that involves persistent pain, fatigue, and other challenging symptoms can have profound implications for emotional health. Here's an exploration of the emotional impact of fibromyalgia:

1. Chronic Pain and Frustration:
   - Persistent Discomfort: Chronic pain is a hallmark of fibromyalgia, impacting different parts of the body. The continuous

discomfort can lead to frustration, irritability, and a sense of helplessness.

- Unpredictability: The unpredictable nature of pain flares and symptom exacerbations can create anxiety and uncertainty, affecting emotional stability.

2. Fatigue and Emotional Exhaustion:

- Constant Fatigue: Fibromyalgia often involves persistent fatigue that can be overwhelming. This physical tiredness contributes to emotional exhaustion, making it challenging to cope with daily stressors.

- Impact on Mood: Prolonged fatigue may lead to mood disturbances, including irritability, sadness, and a sense of being emotionally drained.

3. Impact on Mental Health:

- Depression: Individuals with fibromyalgia have an increased risk of depression. The combination of chronic pain, fatigue, and the challenges of managing a long-term condition can contribute to feelings of hopelessness and sadness.

- Anxiety: Anxiety is another common emotional response. Concerns about the future, uncertainty regarding symptom management, and the impact of fibromyalgia on daily life can contribute to heightened anxiety levels.

4. Social Isolation and Relationship Strain:
   - Limitations on Activities: The physical limitations imposed by fibromyalgia can result in reduced participation in social activities, leading to feelings of isolation and loneliness.
   - Impact on Relationships: Family and social relationships may be strained due to the challenges posed by fibromyalgia. Loved ones may struggle to understand the condition, and the individual may feel a sense of guilt or burden.

5. Cognitive Impairments:
   - Brain Fog: Many individuals with fibromyalgia experience cognitive difficulties often referred to as "fibro fog." This can include memory issues, difficulty concentrating, and mental fatigue,

contributing to frustration and a sense of cognitive decline.

6. Challenges with Self-Identity:
   - Loss of Roles: Fibromyalgia can disrupt various aspects of daily life, leading to a reevaluation of roles and responsibilities. The adjustment to these changes may impact an individual's sense of self-identity and purpose.
   - Emotional Adjustment: Coping with the emotional toll of fibromyalgia often involves a process of emotional adjustment. This may include accepting new limitations, redefining priorities, and finding ways to maintain a positive outlook.

7. Stigma and Misunderstanding:
   - Invisible Illness: Fibromyalgia is often referred to as an "invisible illness" because symptoms are not always apparent to others. This can lead to skepticism, disbelief, or lack of understanding from those who may not grasp the impact of the condition.
   - Stigma: The lack of visible signs may contribute to societal stigma, making it challenging for individuals with

fibromyalgia to receive the understanding and support they need.

8. Coping Strategies and Resilience:
   - Coping Mechanisms: Individuals with fibromyalgia often develop coping mechanisms to navigate the emotional challenges. This may include engaging in activities that bring joy, practicing mindfulness, or seeking support from mental health professionals.
   - Resilience: Despite the emotional toll, many individuals with fibromyalgia demonstrate remarkable resilience. They find ways to adapt, maintain a positive outlook, and continue to pursue a fulfilling life.

Addressing the emotional impact of fibromyalgia involves a holistic approach that integrates medical interventions, emotional support, and coping strategies. Mental health support, including counseling or therapy, can be crucial in helping individuals navigate the emotional complexities associated with fibromyalgia. Additionally, building a strong support network, educating others about the condition, and practicing self-compassion are essential components of emotional well-being for those living with fibromyalgia.

Coping strategies for dealing with stress, anxiety, and depression.

Coping Strategies for Dealing with Stress:

1. Mindfulness and Meditation:
   - Engage in mindfulness practices, such as deep breathing, meditation, or guided imagery, to bring your focus to the present moment and alleviate stress.

2. Regular Exercise:
   - Incorporate regular physical activity into your routine. Exercise helps release endorphins, which act as natural stress relievers.

3. Time Management:
   - Prioritize tasks and break them into manageable steps. Use time-management

techniques to reduce feelings of overwhelm and create a sense of control.

4. Healthy Lifestyle Habits:
  - Maintain a balanced diet, stay hydrated, and ensure adequate sleep. These lifestyle factors play a crucial role in stress management.

5. Social Support:
  - Seek support from friends, family, or a support network. Sharing concerns and feelings can provide emotional relief and perspective.

6. Setting Boundaries:
  - Establish clear boundaries to manage workload and personal commitments. Learning to say no when necessary helps prevent burnout.

7. Relaxation Techniques:
  - Practice relaxation techniques such as progressive muscle relaxation, biofeedback, or aromatherapy to promote a sense of calm.

8. Creative Outlets:

- Engage in creative activities or hobbies that bring you joy. Creative expression can serve as a therapeutic outlet for stress.

Coping Strategies for Dealing with Anxiety:

1. Deep Breathing Exercises:
   - Practice diaphragmatic breathing to calm the nervous system. Inhale deeply through your nose, hold for a moment, and exhale slowly through your mouth.

2. Positive Affirmations:
   - Develop and repeat positive affirmations to counter negative thoughts. Affirmations can shift your mindset and reduce anxiety.

3. Progressive Muscle Relaxation (PMR):
   - Practice PMR to systematically tense and then release different muscle groups, promoting relaxation and reducing physical tension associated with anxiety.

4. Grounding Techniques:
   - Use grounding exercises, such as focusing on sensory experiences or counting

objects in your surroundings, to anchor yourself in the present moment.

5. Cognitive-Behavioral Techniques (CBT):
   - Explore CBT strategies with a therapist to identify and reframe negative thought patterns contributing to anxiety.

6. Regular Exercise:
   - Engage in regular physical activity, as exercise is known to reduce anxiety by promoting the release of endorphins.

7. Limit Caffeine and Sugar Intake:
   - Reduce the consumption of caffeine and sugary foods, as they can contribute to increased nervousness and restlessness.

8. Journaling:
   - Keep a journal to express your thoughts and feelings. Writing can be a therapeutic way to process emotions and gain clarity.

Coping Strategies for Dealing with Depression:

1. Establish Routine:

- Create a daily routine to provide structure and stability. Consistency in activities can be beneficial in managing symptoms of depression.

2. Social Connection:
- Maintain connections with friends and family. Isolation can exacerbate feelings of depression, so seek social support and engage in positive interactions.

3. Set Achievable Goals:
- Break tasks into small, achievable goals. Celebrate accomplishments, no matter how minor, to foster a sense of achievement and purpose.

4. Seek Professional Help:
- Consult with a mental health professional for therapy or counseling. Professional support is crucial for understanding and managing depressive symptoms.

5. Mindfulness and Meditation:
- Practice mindfulness to stay grounded in the present moment. Meditation can help

manage rumination and promote emotional well-being.

6. Engage in Pleasurable Activities:
   - Identify and engage in activities that bring joy and pleasure. This can include hobbies, interests, or spending time in nature.

7. Medication Management:
   - Consult with a healthcare provider to explore medication options if deemed necessary. Antidepressant medications may be prescribed to manage symptoms.

8. Self-Compassion:
   - Practice self-compassion and avoid self-judgment. Understand that dealing with depression is a process, and progress may come in small steps.

Remember that coping strategies may vary among individuals, and it's important to tailor these approaches to your unique needs. If you find that your symptoms persist or worsen, seeking professional help is crucial for comprehensive support and guidance.

Chapter 7: Building a Supportive Community

The importance of a strong support network.

A strong support network is crucial for individuals facing challenges, especially those dealing with chronic conditions like fibromyalgia. Here's an elaboration on the importance of a strong support network:

1. Emotional Support:
   - Validation and Understanding: A support network provides a space where individuals with fibromyalgia feel heard and understood. Emotional validation from friends, family, or support groups helps combat feelings of isolation.

- Empathy and Compassion: Loved ones who understand the emotional impact of fibromyalgia can offer empathy and compassion. This emotional connection is invaluable in navigating the ups and downs of managing a chronic condition.

2. Practical Assistance:
- Help with Daily Tasks: Fibromyalgia can impact physical abilities, making certain daily tasks challenging. A support network that offers practical assistance, whether with household chores, grocery shopping, or transportation, eases the burden on the individual.

- Accommodations and Adaptations: Friends and family can play a crucial role in creating an environment that accommodates the unique needs of someone with fibromyalgia. This may involve making adjustments to living spaces or providing assistance during challenging times.

3. Reducing Social Isolation:
- Connection and Belonging: Fibromyalgia can sometimes lead to social withdrawal due

to symptoms or limitations. A strong support network combats social isolation by fostering a sense of connection and belonging, reducing the impact of loneliness.

- Encouraging Social Activities: Friends and family who actively engage in social activities can motivate individuals with fibromyalgia to participate, promoting a sense of normalcy and enjoyment in shared experiences.

4. Enhancing Mental Health:
- Moral Support: Coping with the emotional toll of fibromyalgia is easier with moral support from loved ones. Having people who offer encouragement, positivity, and reassurance contributes to mental well-being.

- Crisis Intervention: During challenging times or flare-ups, a strong support network provides a safety net for crisis intervention. Knowing that there are people to turn to in times of need can alleviate anxiety and stress.

5. Information and Advocacy:
   - Education and Understanding: A supportive network seeks to educate themselves about fibromyalgia, fostering a deeper understanding of the condition. This knowledge enables friends and family to provide informed support and encouragement.

   - Advocacy: Loved ones can act as advocates, helping individuals with fibromyalgia navigate the healthcare system, communicate effectively with healthcare providers, and ensure their needs are met during medical appointments.

6. Improving Treatment Adherence:
   - Encouragement in Treatment Plans: A supportive network encourages adherence to treatment plans. Whether it involves medication management, physical therapy, or lifestyle changes, knowing that loved ones are invested in their well-being can motivate individuals to follow through with recommended interventions.

- Accompanying to Appointments: Attending medical appointments can be overwhelming, and having someone accompany individuals with fibromyalgia provides emotional support, helps in understanding healthcare instructions, and facilitates better communication with healthcare providers.

7. Promoting Social and Recreational Activities:
   - Participation in Enjoyable Activities: A strong support network actively engages in social and recreational activities that bring joy. Whether it's attending events, going for walks, or enjoying hobbies together, these shared experiences contribute to a positive and fulfilling life.

   - Adaptation of Activities: Friends and family can adapt activities to accommodate the needs of individuals with fibromyalgia, ensuring that they can participate in enjoyable experiences without excessive strain.

In summary, a strong support network plays a central role in the holistic well-being of individuals with fibromyalgia. Beyond practical assistance, emotional support, understanding, and advocacy, the support network becomes a vital source of strength, resilience, and connection. Nurturing and maintaining these relationships contribute significantly to the overall quality of life for individuals living with fibromyalgia.

Guidance on fostering understanding among friends, family, and colleagues.

Fostering understanding about fibromyalgia among friends, family, and colleagues involves effective communication, education, and creating an environment where individuals feel comfortable sharing their experiences. Here's a guide on how to achieve this:

1. Educate Yourself First:
   - Understand Fibromyalgia: Before discussing fibromyalgia with others, ensure

that you have a clear understanding of the condition. Stay informed about its symptoms, impact on daily life, and potential challenges.

2. Choose the Right Time and Place:
   - Select Appropriate Settings: Initiate conversations about fibromyalgia in a comfortable and private setting where there's enough time for discussion. This ensures that the information is conveyed in a relaxed and focused environment.

3. Use Clear and Simple Language:
   - Avoid Medical Jargon: Explain fibromyalgia using clear and simple language, avoiding medical jargon that might be confusing. Use relatable examples to help others grasp the impact of the condition.

4. Share Personal Experiences:
   - Express Your Feelings: Share your personal experiences with fibromyalgia, expressing how it affects your daily life. Emphasize both the physical and emotional aspects of living with the condition.

- Highlight Challenges: Discuss specific challenges you face, such as fatigue, pain, and cognitive difficulties. Providing concrete examples helps others relate to your experiences.

5. Provide Educational Resources:
- Share Reliable Information: Offer educational resources, such as pamphlets, articles, or reputable websites, that provide accurate information about fibromyalgia. This allows individuals to learn more at their own pace.

6. Encourage Questions and Open Dialogue:
- Invite Questions: Create an open and non-judgmental space for questions. Encourage friends, family, and colleagues to ask about fibromyalgia, fostering a two-way dialogue.

- Address Misconceptions: Be prepared to address any misconceptions or myths about fibromyalgia. Clarify information to enhance understanding and dispel common misconceptions.

7. Emphasize the Variable Nature of Symptoms:

   - Highlight Variability: Emphasize that symptoms of fibromyalgia can vary from day to day. Help others understand that what may be manageable one day could be more challenging on another.

8. Communicate Treatment Strategies:

   - Discuss Treatment Approaches: Share information about the treatment strategies you are using, whether it involves medications, lifestyle changes, or alternative therapies. Explain how these approaches contribute to symptom management.

9. Express Specific Needs for Support:

   - Communicate Your Needs: Clearly express the type of support that would be helpful. Whether it's understanding during flare-ups, assistance with certain tasks, or emotional support, letting others know your needs fosters a supportive environment.

10. Involve Loved Ones in Healthcare Visits:

- Invite Participation: Encourage friends or family members to join you during healthcare visits. This involvement allows them to gain insights from healthcare professionals and ask questions directly.

11. Engage in Joint Activities:
   - Participate Together: Engage in joint activities that raise awareness about fibromyalgia, such as attending support group meetings or events organized by fibromyalgia advocacy organizations.

12. Model Open Communication:
   - Demonstrate Openness: Be open about how fibromyalgia impacts your daily life. By modeling transparent communication, you create an environment where others feel comfortable sharing their thoughts and concerns.

13. Provide Updates on Your Condition:
   - Regularly Communicate: Keep friends, family, and colleagues updated on your condition. Sharing updates allows them to better understand the ongoing nature of

fibromyalgia and how it may evolve over time.

14. Express Gratitude:
  - Acknowledge Support: Express gratitude for the support you receive. Acknowledge the efforts made by friends, family, and colleagues to understand and assist you in managing fibromyalgia.

By fostering understanding through open communication, education, and shared experiences, you create a supportive network that enhances the overall well-being of individuals with fibromyalgia. Building this understanding is an ongoing process that strengthens relationships and promotes a more compassionate and inclusive environment.

Chapter 8: Patient Perspectives

Personal stories from individuals living with fibromyalgia.

Sarah Saxe

Meet Sarah, a resilient individual living with fibromyalgia. Her journey is a testament to strength, adaptability, and the power of a positive mindset.

Sarah was a vibrant professional, dedicated to her demanding job in marketing. However, her life took an unexpected turn when she started experiencing persistent pain, fatigue, and cognitive difficulties. After numerous doctor visits and tests, she received a diagnosis of fibromyalgia.

Initially, Sarah felt overwhelmed and frustrated. The unpredictable nature of her symptoms made it challenging to plan her work and personal life. Daily tasks that were once routine became sources of discomfort, and the vibrant energy she once had seemed elusive.

Amidst the adjustments and uncertainties, Sarah decided to take charge of her well-being. She began by educating herself about fibromyalgia, learning about symptom management, lifestyle changes, and the importance of a holistic approach to health. Armed with knowledge, she set realistic goals for herself, acknowledging the need for both professional and personal adjustments.

Work became a collaborative effort. Sarah initiated an open conversation with her supervisor, explaining the impact of fibromyalgia on her productivity and proposing a flexible work schedule. Together, they crafted a plan that allowed her to work from home when needed and provided breaks during the day to manage fatigue.

Sarah embraced a comprehensive treatment plan. Regular medical check-ups and consultations with specialists became integral parts of her routine. Medication, prescribed by her healthcare team, helped alleviate some symptoms, and she actively participated in physical therapy sessions to maintain mobility and manage pain.

Understanding the importance of emotional well-being, Sarah prioritized self-care. She incorporated mindfulness and meditation into her daily routine, creating moments of tranquility amidst life's challenges. Journaling became a therapeutic outlet, helping her process emotions and track patterns in her symptoms.

Sarah's social support network played a vital role in her journey. She openly communicated with family and friends, explaining the intricacies of fibromyalgia and expressing her needs. Loved ones responded with empathy, providing practical assistance when required and offering emotional support during tougher times.

Recognizing the benefits of staying active, Sarah engaged in tailored exercise routines.

Low-impact activities, such as swimming and gentle yoga, became her allies in managing pain and maintaining overall well-being. She embraced the concept of pacing, learning to listen to her body and adjust her activities accordingly.

Sarah's journey wasn't without challenges. There were days when fatigue and pain tested her resolve. Yet, she remained resilient, drawing strength from her support network, adjusting her strategies as needed, and celebrating the small victories along the way.

In her personal ordeal, Sarah discovered the power of adaptation and the importance of self-advocacy. Her positive mindset, combined with a proactive approach to her health, allowed her to lead a fulfilling life despite the challenges of fibromyalgia. Her story serves as a motivation for real-life patients, showing that with resilience, education, and a strong support system, it's possible to navigate the complexities of fibromyalgia and continue to thrive.

David Samuels

Meet David, a resilient individual on his journey with fibromyalgia. His story reflects the diverse experiences and challenges that individuals with this condition may face.

David was a passionate teacher who loved engaging with his students and exploring innovative teaching methods. However, his life took an unexpected turn when he started experiencing chronic pain, fatigue, and cognitive difficulties. The relentless symptoms became overwhelming, prompting David to seek medical help.

After a series of consultations and medical tests, David received the diagnosis of fibromyalgia. This revelation initially left him feeling disheartened and uncertain about his future in education. However, David was determined not to let fibromyalgia define him or limit his ability to make a positive impact on his students.

Facing the challenges head-on, David engaged in open communication with his school administration and colleagues. He shared insights into fibromyalgia, educating them about the condition's impact on his daily life. Together, they explored ways to make adjustments to his work environment, such as providing ergonomic seating and allowing flexible work hours during flare-ups.

Embracing a multidisciplinary approach to his health, David collaborated with various healthcare professionals. His treatment plan included a combination of medication, physical therapy, and counseling to address both the physical and emotional aspects of fibromyalgia. He actively participated in support groups, finding solace in connecting with others who shared similar experiences.

Understanding the importance of maintaining a work-life balance, David integrated self-care practices into his routine. He established a consistent sleep schedule, engaged in mindfulness meditation, and adopted a balanced diet to support his overall well-being. These lifestyle adjustments, though initially challenging, became essential components of David's resilience against the impact of fibromyalgia.

One of David's greatest sources of strength was his support network. His family and friends rallied around him, offering encouragement and practical assistance during periods of increased symptom severity. Colleagues stepped in to share the workload, fostering a collaborative and understanding work environment.

David's journey with fibromyalgia wasn't without its hurdles. There were moments of frustration and fatigue that tested his resolve. Yet, through persistence and a positive mindset, he continued to pursue his passion for teaching. David embraced adaptive teaching methods, incorporating technology and collaborative learning to enhance his students' experience.

In sharing his story, David became an advocate for fibromyalgia awareness within the education community. He participated in workshops and seminars, educating fellow educators about the condition and fostering a more inclusive and supportive environment for those facing similar challenges.

David's journey exemplifies the resilience and determination that individuals with fibromyalgia can demonstrate. By adapting and proactively addressing the unique challenges posed by the condition, he continued to thrive in his profession and make a meaningful impact on the lives of his students. His story serves as an inspiration for others facing fibromyalgia, showcasing the possibilities of living a fulfilling life despite the complexities of the condition.

Insights into their unique challenges, triumphs, and coping mechanisms.

Insights into Sarah's Journey:

Unique Challenges:
  - Professional Adaptation: Sarah faced the challenge of adapting her professional life to accommodate the unpredictable nature of fibromyalgia symptoms. Negotiating a

flexible work schedule and finding ways to manage her workload were essential adjustments.

- Balancing Self-Care: Balancing self-care with work commitments posed a challenge. Sarah had to prioritize her well-being while fulfilling professional responsibilities, requiring careful planning and effective communication with her supervisor.

- Emotional Resilience: Navigating the emotional impact of fibromyalgia, including frustration and the need for ongoing adjustments, required significant emotional resilience. Coping with the emotional toll of a chronic condition became an integral aspect of her journey.

Triumphs:
- Professional Collaboration: Sarah's triumph lay in successfully collaborating with her supervisor to create a work environment that supported her needs. This collaboration showcased the possibility of maintaining professional success while managing fibromyalgia.

- Holistic Well-Being: Sarah's commitment to a holistic approach to well-being, incorporating physical, emotional, and lifestyle aspects, led to triumphs in symptom management and overall quality of life.

- Support Network Strength: Building a robust support network played a pivotal role in Sarah's triumphs. Open communication and shared understanding within her support circle contributed to her resilience.

Coping Mechanisms:
- Educational Empowerment: Sarah coped by educating herself about fibromyalgia, empowering her to make informed decisions about treatment options, lifestyle changes, and self-care practices.

- Mindfulness Practices: Incorporating mindfulness and meditation into her daily routine became a crucial coping mechanism. These practices provided moments of calm amidst the challenges, contributing to her emotional well-being.

- Celebrating Small Victories: Sarah's coping strategy included celebrating small victories. Recognizing and acknowledging achievements, no matter how minor, became a positive reinforcement in her journey.

Insights into David's Journey:

Unique Challenges:
- Adaptation in Teaching Methods: David faced the challenge of adapting his teaching methods to accommodate the physical and cognitive challenges posed by fibromyalgia. Embracing innovative and adaptive teaching approaches became essential.

- Advocacy in the Education Community: Advocating for fibromyalgia awareness within the education community presented a unique challenge. David took on the responsibility of educating colleagues about the condition and fostering a more inclusive environment.

- Managing Work-Life Balance: Balancing the demands of teaching with self-care and

symptom management was a continual
challenge. David had to find effective ways
to maintain his passion for teaching while
prioritizing his health.

Triumphs:
  - Collaborative Work Environment:
David's triumph lay in fostering a
collaborative work environment where
colleagues supported his needs and students
benefited from innovative teaching methods.
This showcased the possibility of thriving in
a professional setting despite fibromyalgia.

  - Educational Advocacy: Becoming an
advocate for fibromyalgia awareness within
the education community was a significant
triumph. David's efforts contributed to
creating a more informed and supportive
environment for educators facing similar
challenges.

  - Inclusive Teaching Practices:
Implementing inclusive teaching practices
that accommodated both his needs and the
diverse learning styles of his students was a
triumph. David's adaptive teaching methods

showcased the importance of flexibility in education.

Coping Mechanisms:
- Multidisciplinary Healthcare Approach: David coped by actively engaging in a multidisciplinary healthcare approach. Regular consultations with healthcare professionals, including physical therapy and counseling, played a crucial role in his overall well-being.

- Support Network Engagement: Building and engaging with a strong support network was a coping mechanism for David. His family, friends, and colleagues provided emotional support and practical assistance during challenging times.

- Adaptive Teaching Strategies: David's coping strategies included embracing adaptive teaching strategies. Incorporating technology, collaborative learning, and innovative approaches allowed him to continue pursuing his passion for teaching while managing fibromyalgia.

These insights into Sarah and David's journeys highlight the diverse challenges, triumphs, and coping mechanisms associated with living with fibromyalgia. Each individual's approach to their unique journey showcases the resilience and adaptability that can be integral in navigating the complexities of a chronic condition.

Chapter 9: Looking Forward: Research and Hope

Encouragement for individuals to stay informed, hopeful, and engaged in their healthcare journey.

Staying informed, hopeful, and engaged in your healthcare journey is crucial for individuals facing health challenges, including conditions like fibromyalgia. Here's an elaboration on the encouragement to maintain an active role in your healthcare:

1. Knowledge Empowers:
   - Understanding Your Condition: Staying informed about your health condition, such

as fibromyalgia, empowers you to actively participate in decisions regarding your care. Knowledge about symptoms, treatment options, and self-management strategies allows you to make informed choices alongside your healthcare team.

- Advocating for Yourself: Being well-informed transforms you into an effective advocate for your health. It enables you to communicate more effectively with healthcare professionals, ask pertinent questions, and actively participate in discussions about your treatment plan.

2. Hope as a Driving Force:
- Embracing Positivity: Maintaining hope is a powerful force that positively influences your mental and emotional well-being. Recognize that medical science is continuously advancing, and breakthroughs in treatments or management strategies for conditions like fibromyalgia may occur.

- Focusing on Progress: Celebrate small victories and progress on your healthcare journey. Whether it's finding a treatment that alleviates some symptoms, improving daily functioning, or receiving support from your network, acknowledging these positive aspects contributes to a hopeful outlook.

3. Active Engagement Yields Benefits:
   - Collaborating with Healthcare Professionals: Actively engaging with your healthcare team fosters a collaborative relationship. Share your experiences, concerns, and preferences openly. This collaboration enhances the effectiveness of your treatment plan and ensures that it aligns with your unique needs.

   - Participating in Lifestyle Modifications: Engage actively in lifestyle modifications recommended by your healthcare team. This might include exercise, dietary changes, stress management, and sleep hygiene. Your commitment to these aspects significantly contributes to the overall success of your healthcare plan.

4. Building a Support Network:
   - Connecting with Others: Engage with individuals facing similar health challenges.

Whether through support groups, online communities, or local events, connecting with others provides a sense of community and shared understanding. Exchanging experiences and insights can be both comforting and informative.

- Involving Loved Ones: Your healthcare journey is not solely an individual effort. Involve your loved ones, sharing your goals, challenges, and triumphs with them. Their support can be invaluable, providing emotional strength and encouragement.

5. Adapting to Changes:
- Flexibility in Approaches: Understand that healthcare journeys often involve adjustments. Be flexible in your approach to treatment plans, lifestyle modifications, and coping strategies. Embracing adaptability allows you to navigate changes effectively.

- Acknowledging Progression: Recognize that health conditions may have varying trajectories. Staying engaged means acknowledging and addressing changes in your health status promptly, seeking guidance from your healthcare team as needed.

6. Seeking Emotional Support:

- Mental Health Matters: Prioritize your mental health by seeking emotional support. This can include talking to a therapist, counselor, or mental health professional who can provide guidance in managing the emotional aspects of your healthcare journey.

- Family and Friends: Lean on your support network of family and friends during challenging times. Open communication about your needs and feelings fosters understanding and strengthens the emotional bonds that contribute to overall well-being.

In conclusion, encouragement for individuals to stay informed, hopeful, and engaged in their healthcare journey emphasizes the transformative power of knowledge, optimism, and active involvement. By embracing these principles, individuals can navigate their healthcare journey with resilience, foster positive outcomes, and enhance their overall quality of life.

Printed in Great Britain
by Amazon

36670884R00057